EAT YOURSELF SKINNY

30 DELICIOUS SUPERFOOD SALAD RECIPES TO REV YOUR METABOLISM AND MAKE FAT CRY!

Includes 30 Satisfying, Anti-Inflammatory, Antioxidant-Rich Recipes Under 400 Calories to Promote Weight Loss, Increase Energy and Boost Your Metabolism

Disclaimer

The information in this book is not to be used as medical advice. The recipes should be used in combination with guidance from your physician. Please consult your physician before beginning any diet. It is especially important for those with diabetes, and those on medications to consult with their physician before making changes to their diet.

Disclaimer and Terms of Use: Effort has been made to ensure that the information in this book is accurate and complete, however, the author and the publisher do not warrant the accuracy of the information, text and graphics contained within the book due to the rapidly changing nature of science, research, known and unknown facts and internet. The Author and the publisher do not hold any responsibility for errors, omissions or contrary interpretation of the subject matter herein. This book is presented solely for motivational and informational purposes only.

Introduction

Eat Yourself Skinny: 30 Delicious Superfood Salad Recipes to Rev Your Metabolism and Make Fat Cry! Introduces the holy grail of any diet plan: the Superfood. Superfoods swoop into your preservative-rich land of Oreos and potato chips to take hold of your digestion and metabolism once again. A superfood represents any nutritive-dense, low-calorie food that stands out amongst the other vegetables and fruits. The superfood is prominent in its dense antioxidant packaging, in its provision of complete proteins, and in its elaborate assistance to your well-being.

Thousands of years ago in various environments around the world, our ancestors worked to survive with the benefits of their local superfood. They nourished and protected themselves from the harsh environment with the nutrient-packed fruits and vegetables and seeds they could find. For example, the quinoa seed was essential in the survival of the Andes people while the Noni fruit fought off E-coli on Polynesian islands.

The wealth of these enriched superfoods can be yours with these essential salad recipes. The recipes in this book are split into three sections: the Green Superfoods, the Fruit and Nut Superfoods, and the Seed Superfoods. Each category promotes a different nourishing, weight-loss element. Look to each category to put a boost of protein and antioxidants in your daily life. Assist your brain and digestive tract in proper function with the anti-inflammatory elements. And allow your thyroid gland to emit correct weight-regulatory hormones with honed cell-to-cell communication via the Seed Superfood Omega 3 fatty acids.

Each salad yields less than four hundred calories of nutrient-dense foods. These super salads are all you need to build a happy, healthy lifestyle. In addition, these superfood super salads can be eaten as a lunch replacement for your typical hamburger and fries, or they can be eaten as a snack when you just feel like having something extra nutritious and tasty. And if you're craving something sweet but don't want to compromise your diet with another sugary dessert, try the Tropical Coconut Fruit Salad or the Polynesian Noni Fruit Salad; it's guaranteed they'll satisfy your sweet tooth!

Enjoy!
Kasia

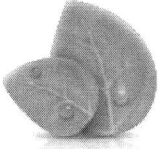 # SUPERFOODS

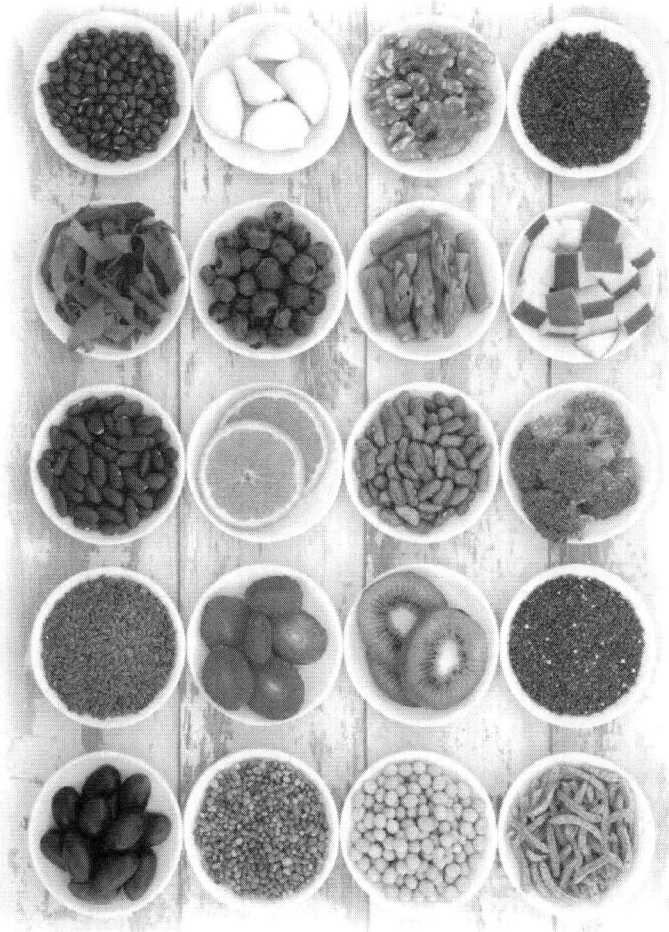

Table of Contents

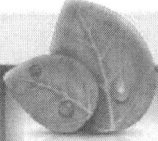

GREEN SUPERFOODS
SKINNY SALADS

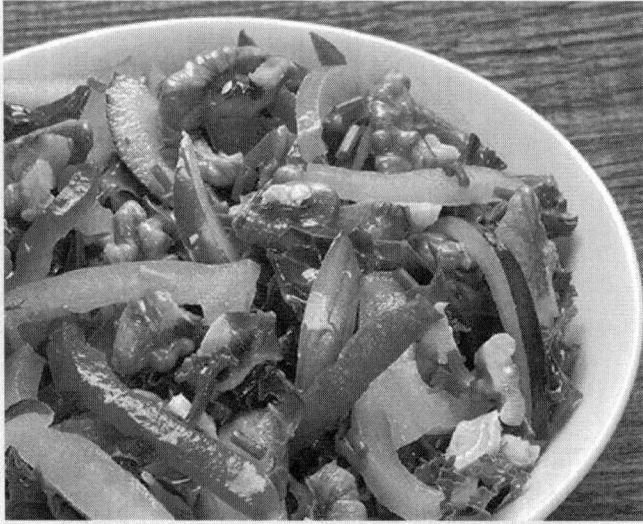

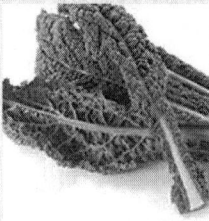

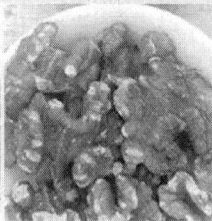

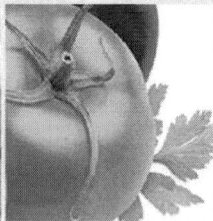

Green Superfood Skinny Salads

After hammering the Food Guide Pyramid into your brain, searching for answers to that ultimate loss-weight question, you think you've got it down: green vegetables. Yes. You know to eat your green vegetables, to incorporate salads into your diet in order to maintain brain and muscle and gut capability. Furthermore, green vegetables provide fiber and adequate energy at a low caloric cost. You sit back with your celery stick and wait for your waist to disappear.

There's a trick to this, however. In order to maximize your green vegetable munching, you must hone in on precise mean, Green Superfoods. Green Superfoods are, of course, low in calories. All you needed to know, right? But there's more. Compared to other green vegetables, Green Superfoods boast many more digestible nutrients. Therefore, nothing slips through the cracks of your system because your digestive tract can't handle complex, plant-based nature. Green Superfoods also contain vast amounts of vitamins and minerals that aid in cell protection and eventual healing. Furthermore, Green Superfoods contain muscle-maintaining proteins and gut-healthy bacteria.

Green Superfoods also maintain proper brain function in their maintenance of hemoglobin in your blood. In order for your neurons to properly fire in your brain, your heart must pump adequate amounts of blood into your brain. The more oxygen via your blood and into your brain, the more alert and ready you are to make decisions. Green Superfoods also contain the pigment, chlorophyll. This is the element that allows these plants to maintain their rich, green color. The structure of the chlorophyll is fascinating in that it resembles hemoglobin, those oxygen-rich cells flowing in your bloodstream. If you eat more of these chlorophyll-filled Green Superfoods, your body will begin to produce more hemoglobin. And, therefore, your brain and the rest of your body will be filled with a boost of oxygen. Be prepared to wake up!

KALE

Kale is often an overlooked Green Superfood. Something like three thousand years ago, however, numerous Celtic tribes took advantage of kale's nutritional benefits, fiber, phytochemicals, and flavonoids. Kale has caught up to us in this millennium, producing cancer prevention in the way of its phytochemicals and reducing cell inflammation with forty-five different flavonoids.

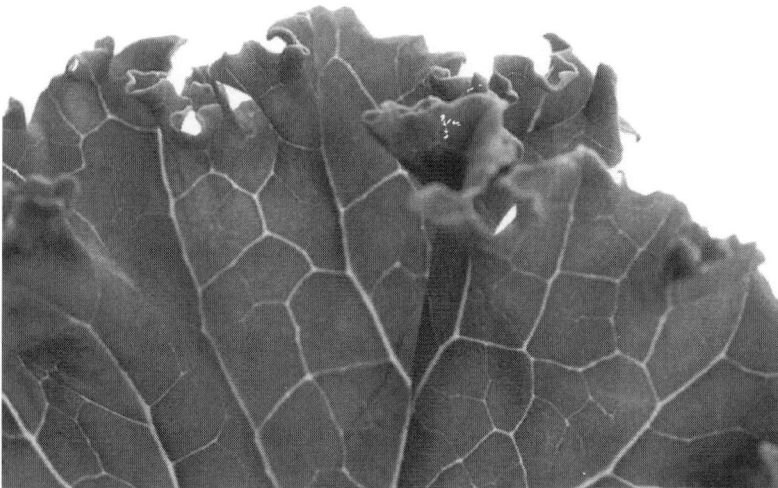

Pecorino Walnut-Topped Kale Salad

Makes 4-6 servings.

Ingredients:
½ cup walnut pieces
¼ cup golden raisins
1 tbsp. white wine vinegar
1 tbsp. water
¼ cup panko
1 minced garlic clove
Dash of kosher salt
3 tbsp. olive oil
14 ounces Tuscan Kale, washed
2 ounces pecorino cheese, grated
Half a lemon, juiced
Ground black pepper to taste

Directions:
Begin by preparing your walnuts. You'll want to preheat the oven to 350 degrees Fahrenheit. Lay out your walnuts evenly on a baking sheet in a single layer. Bake them for ten minutes. After the walnuts cool, chop them into salad-topping pieces.

Prepare your raisins in a saucepan with white wine vinegar and water; heat on low for about five minutes. Set the raisins aside, remaining in the vinegar.

Toast your panko, your minced garlic, and 2 tsp. olive oil in a skillet until your panko emotes a golden color. Set the panko aside.

Trim your kale and remove the center ribs. Stack your leaves and roll them into tubes. Cut them crosswise into tiny ribbons.

Place your pre-cut kale into a large salad bowl. Toss on your pre-grated pecorino, walnuts, and vinegar raisins. You can sprinkle the simmered vinegar atop as well. Add the rest of the olive oil—2 tbsp. and half a lemon's worth of juice. Toss the kale salad, allowing the toppings to reposition. Adjust your seasonings as you please with salt and ground pepper. Immediately prior to serving, add the garlic panko. Enjoy your vibrant phytochemical-rich kale salad!

Fiber-Stocked Warm Kale Salad With A Balsamic Glaze

Makes 4-6 Servings.

Ingredients:
2 tbsp. butter
¼ cup chopped onion
1 chopped red pepper
1 chopped yellow pepper
8 ounces sliced Portobello mushrooms
4 cups kale
1 tsp. minced garlic
1 tbsp. balsamic vinegar
¼ cup Asiago cheese
Salt and pepper to taste

Directions:
Prepare one large skillet over a medium-heated burner; melt one tablespoon of butter. Toss in your pre-chopped onions, red pepper, and yellow pepper. Sautee the vegetables in the butter until they are soft. Next, add the remaining one tablespoon of butter to the skillet. Toss your sliced portabellas in there, as well. Sautee for another several minutes until your vegetables are browned.

Prepare your kale appropriately; remove the ribs and chop in diagonals across the leaves to create smaller pieces. Add the kale to the pre-sauteed, pre-heated skillet. Add the minced garlic and the balsamic vinegar, as well. Continue to sautee the mixture until your kale is a dark green. Do not allow your kale to wilt.

Remove the skillet from the heat and top the salad with Asiago cheese, salt, and pepper. Enjoy your heated, low-calorie salad complete with the fiber and added antioxidants of a kale-rich diet.

SPINACH

Spinach packs a ton of Vitamin K and A in each serving. It's also swimming with manganese, folic acid, dietary fiber, calcium, and protein. Protein, of course, is a muscle-building, hunger-averting element of your every day diet. Folic acid is essential, as well, as it provides antioxidants, essential for reduced cell inflammation. Spinach is incredibly low in calories, boasting a mere seven calories per cup. It is a wonderful Superfood, easily based in any afternoon salad.

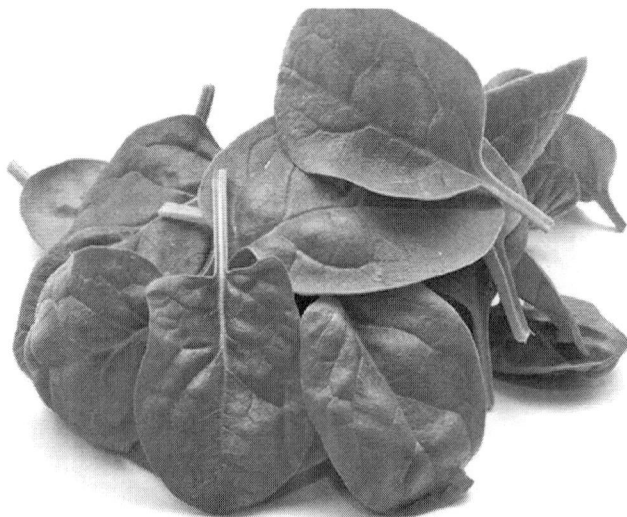

Cran-Almond Manganese-Stocked Spinach Salad

Makes 4-6 Servings.

Ingredients:
1 tbsp. butter
¾ cup almonds, slivered
1 pound spinach, bite-sized pieces
1 cup dried cranberries
2 tbsp. poppy seeds
1 tbsp. sesame seeds
½ cup coconut sugar
2 tsp. diced onion
¼ tsp. paprika
¼ cup white wine vinegar
¼ cup apple cider vinegar
½ cup vegetable oil

Directions:
Melt the tablespoon of butter in a medium-sized saucepan over medium heat. Add the ¾ cup almonds, stirring until the almonds are toasted. Remove them from the heat prior to slicing.

To the side, whisk sesame seeds, poppy seeds, sugar, diced onion, paprika, white wine vinegar, apple cider vinegar, and your vegetable oil together. Add this mixture to a large bowl and toss in the spinach, allowing the ingredients to mix appropriately. Prior to serving, add your sliced, toasted almonds and dried cranberries. Enjoy!

Poppy Seed-Drizzled Avocado Strawberry Spinach Salad

Makes 2-4 Servings.

Ingredients

Salad:
6 cups baby spinach
1 pint sliced strawberries
1 diced avocado
4 ounces gorgonzola
¼ cup toasted and sliced almonds
1 sliced red onion

Poppy Seed Dressing:
½ cup avocado oil
3 tbsp. apple cider vinegar
2 tbsp. honey
1 tbsp. poppy seeds
Salt and pepper to taste

Directions:
Prepare your almonds by preheating the oven to 350 degrees Fahrenheit. Align them on a baking sheet evenly, in a single layer, and bake for ten minutes. Set them aside, allowing them to cool, prior to slicing them.

Toss all the salad ingredients together in a large bowl, allowing the ingredients to distribute accordingly.

Whisk the poppy seed dressing ingredients together in a medium sized bowl. Add salt and pepper to taste. Serve with the prepared salad.

Beet with Heat Spinach Salad

Makes 4-6 Servings.

Ingredients:
8 cups spinach
1 tbsp. olive oil
1 cup sliced onion
2 chopped tomatoes
2 tbsp. olives
2 tbsp. chopped parsley
1 minced garlic clove
2 cups sliced and steamed beets
2 tbsp. balsamic vinegar
¼ tsp. salt
¼ tsp. pepper

Directions:
Set your spinach in a large salad bowl.

Heat the olive oil in a skillet over medium heat. Toss in your onion and stir for approximately two minutes. Next, add your tomatoes, olives, parsley, and garlic. Stir over medium heat until the tomatoes lose their proper consistency. Next, add the beets, the vinegar, and the salt and pepper. Take the mixture off the heat after two more minutes.

Toss the beet mixture with the spinach leaves and serve warm.

ARTICHOKES

That pine-cone-looking green thing in the vegetable aisle: that's an artichoke. And it's a mean weapon residing in your Green Superfood power group. It's filled with fiber and Vitamin C; Vitamin C is an important proponent in relieving stress as it dramatically decreases the hormone cortisol. When cortisol is running amok in your brain for too long, it begins to actually kill brain cells in your hippocampus; your hippocampus is the part of the brain that allows short-term memories to convert to long-term memories. The hippocampus is also responsible for the creation of new brain cells. Therefore, a hearty dose of Vitamin C via Green Superfood the artichoke is beneficial for brain health and body health. When cooked and thrown into salads, the artichoke provides a tasty, wonderful texture. Furthermore, it's a wonderful weight loss tool; it packs only forty-seven calories in each medium-sized artichoke.

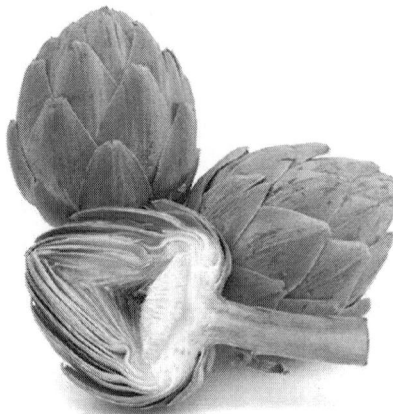

Vitamin C-Boosting Artichoke Tomato Salad

Makes 4-5 Servings.

Ingredients:
5 large chopped tomatoes
¼ tsp. salt
¼ tsp. pepper
7 ounces marinated and quartered artichoke hearts
1/3 cup sliced Kalamata olives
2 tbsp. minced parsley
2 tbsp. white wine vinegar
2 minced garlic cloves

Directions:
Prepare your tomatoes by chopping them into medium-sized wedges. Arrange the five chopped tomatoes on your salad platter and sprinkle them with salt and pepper.

Place your marinated artichoke hearts, olives, parsley, vinegar, and your minced garlic cloves in a medium-sized bowl and toss. Allow the ingredients to distribute properly.

Prior to serving, spoon the artichoke mixture overtop the tomato platter. Enjoy this nutrient-rich platter of artichoke and tomato goodness.

Stress-Relieving Bean and Artichoke Salad

Makes 2-4 Servings.

Ingredients:
3 cups white beans
½ can artichoke hearts
2/3 cup diced green pepper
1/3 cup chopped black olives
¼ cup chopped red onion
¼ cup chopped parsley
¼ ounce chopped mint leaves
¾ tsp. dried basil
1/3 cup olive oil
¼ cup red wine vinegar
Salt and pepper to taste

Directions:
Toss everything—your vegetables and your beans and your leaves—in a large salad bowl. Combine the olive oil and the vinegar in a jar and shake. Pour the mixture overtop the salad and stir, allowing the glaze to coat the vegetables. Allow to chill overnight prior to serving.

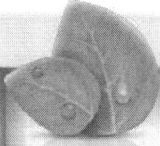

GREEN SUPERFOODS

SALAD DRESSINGS AND GLAZE

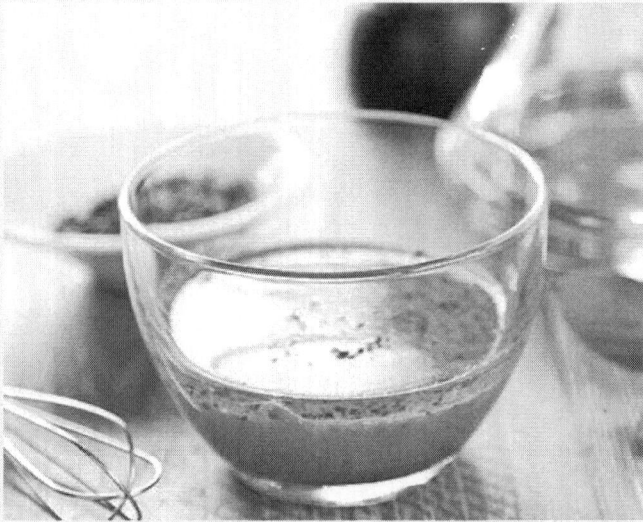

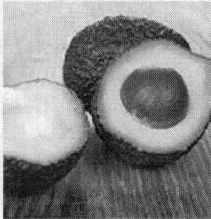 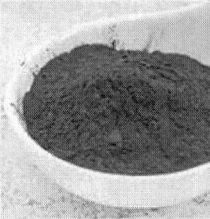 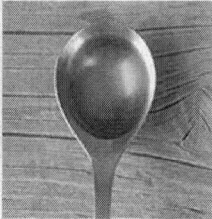

WHEATGRASS

The real goodness of wheat occurs outside the realms of breads and pastas. Allow whole grain seeds to sprout into wheat grass. Wheat grass is the nutritional antithesis to whole grains in that it provides essential nutrients and is void of gluten, a protein composite that disagrees with millions of people's digestive tracts.

Wheat grass contains an alkaline component that boosts healthy blood. Furthermore, it is incredibly beneficial for weight loss: any irritation or disruption in your thyroid gland is normalized with the existence of wheat grass. A proper-functioning thyroid gland promotes weight loss and body cleansing. Wheatgrass comes in powdered forms found in your local grocery store or any natural health food store.

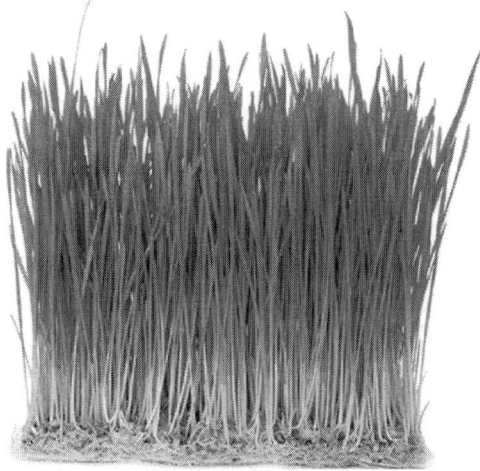

Essential Wheatgrass Ranch Salad Dressing/Dip

Makes 2-4 Servings.

Ingredients:
1 scoop organic wheatgrass powder
¾ cup extra virgin olive oil
¼ cup lemon juice
2 tbsp. wheat-free tamari
1 and ¼ cup filtered water
½ cup soaked sunflower seeds
1 cup hemp seeds
1 tsp. garlic or 1 small clove
1 tbsp. chopped jalapeño, seeded
¾ tsp. sea salt
¼ tsp. black pepper
1 tbsp. dried dill
¼ cup fresh parsley
¼ cup fresh cilantro

Blend all ingredients in the blender on high for 30 seconds or until you reach a creamy consistency. Chill and serve with any kale or spinach salad for a zesty, overarching, healthy flavor or as a dip with your favorite vegetables. This dressing is truly yummy!

Garlic Wheatgrass Salad Glaze

Makes 2-4 Servings.

Ingredients:
1 large avocado
2/3 cup filtered water
4 crushed garlic cloves
8 tbsp. fresh lemon juice
2 tbsp. apple cider vinegar
1 tsp. ginger powder
1 scoop organic wheatgrass powder
1 tsp. thyme
Salt and pepper to taste

Directions:
Toss the above ingredients into a high-capacity blender. Blend until the glaze is smooth. Drizzle the dressing onto any fresh Green Superfood salad for a weight-loss boost.

WILD BLUE-GREEN ALGAE

Reconsider your pre-diagnosis of what algae are. You think of it as the stuff growing rampant in your fish bowl or the stuff floating at the top of a brown man-made lake. Disgusting. But the wild blue-green algae are actually some of the most powerful foods known to man. It's sixty percent protein—elbowing out even the most protein-stocked steaks. Its remarkable amount of B vitamins and chlorophyll also maintain muscle mass and help to repair your hippocampus, the part of the brain responsible for memories.

SPIRULINA, A TYPE OF WILD BLUE-GREEN ALGAE

Thousands of years ago, people of what is now Mexico and Africa looked to the spirulina micro-algae for one of the best protein sources; it contains seventy percent protein. These days, it is utilized as an excellent weight loss supplement; it reduces cravings and halts blood sugar spikes in their tracks.

Like the Wheatgrass, Blue-Green Algae and, therefore, Spirulina, must be eaten via powders. The powders have all the appropriate nutrients the blue-green algae boasts in easily digestible forms.

Mean Green Avocado Spirulina Salad Dressing

Serves 2.

Ingredients:
½ diced avocado
1 tsp. spirulina powder of choice (Oriya organics works well)
1 small chopped zucchini
¼ cup hemp seeds
1 tbsp. mellow white miso
2 tbsp. lemon juice
½ cup filtered water

Directions:
Toss all the ingredients into a high-action blender and blend. The dressing should be smooth, not chunky. Add salt and pepper to taste and add the protein-rich goodness to any leafy green salad of choice for the added Superfood benefits.

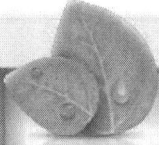

FRESH FRUIT AND NUT SUPERFOOD

SKINNY SALADS

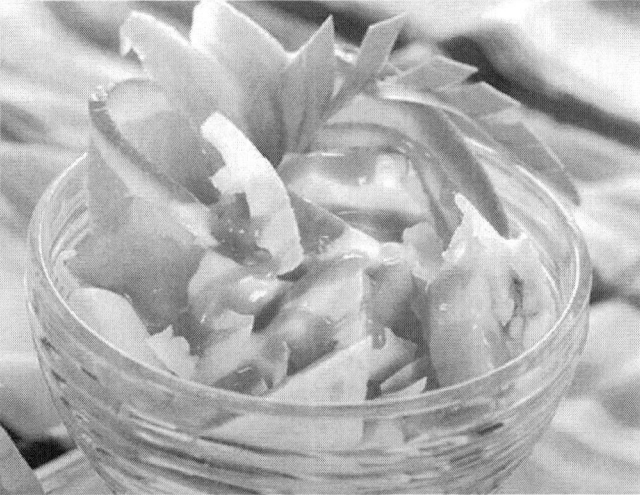

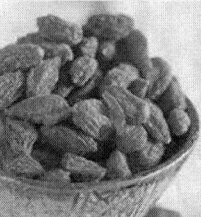

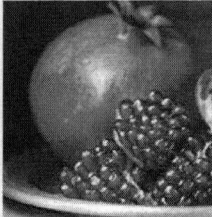

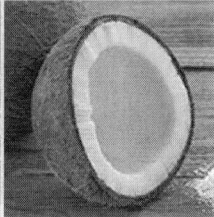

Fresh Fruit and Nut Superfood Skinny Salads

If you ache with a sweet tooth, look to the natural sweet elements of the Fruit and Nut Superfoods. Fruit and Nut Superfoods provide an over-arching boost of antioxidants. Antioxidants sound great—their existence is touted throughout the aisles at your local grocery. But what are they, exactly?

To understand antioxidants, you must first understand free radicals. Free radicals are formed as a product of various chemical reactions in your body. These chemical reactions are necessary in order to proceed with proper functions; for example, every time a neurotransmitter ascends through your brain networks, the communication between cells emits a free radical. Unfortunately, our free radical load has been increasing over the years with the existence of second hand cigarette smoke, any burnt barbecue foods, radiation, and deep fried fair foods. Was that deep fried Twinkie really worth it? With the build up of free radicals in your system, proper communication between cells is simply nonexistent. Free radicals cause inflammation in each neuron, and in each stomach lining and blood cell.

Fortunately, antioxidants swoop in from these Fruit and Nut Superfoods and decrease inflammation, allowing enhanced communication throughout your body. Enhanced communication allows for a healthy immune system; therefore, antioxidants allow you to escape from the onset of colds and flus.

POMEGRANATE

Look to the vibrant Pomegranate for a boost of rich antioxidants. Pomegranate has been the underlying ingredient of many Indian health remedies for thousands of years. Beyond its shot of antioxidants, it fuels you with vitamin C and potassium. Research suggests it lowers blood pressure and decreases plaque build up on your arteries.

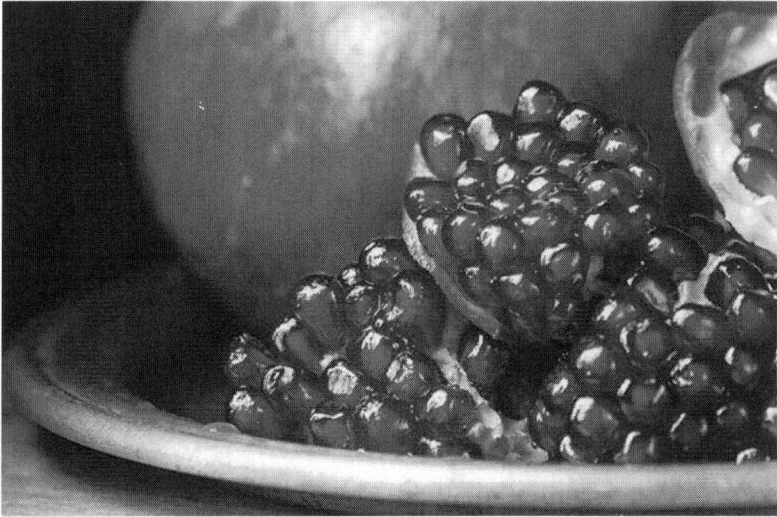

Winter Passion Pomegranate Fruit Salad

Makes 2-4 Servings.

Ingredients:
1 pomegranate
2 oranges
2 grapefruits
2 apples
1 pear
1 tbsp. coconut sugar

Directions:
Slice your pomegranates in half. Squeeze the two halves' juices and seeds into a large salad bowl. Remove as much membrane as you can from the two halves. Add slices of both oranges and grapefruit to the large salad bowl. Squeeze out the remaining juice from each membrane, as well. Slice the apples and pears and toss them into the large bowl. Pour the tablespoon of coconut sugar into the fruit bowl and toss well to coat the fruit. Enjoy your antioxidant-rich fruit bowl!

Pomegranate Persimmon Layered Salad

Makes 1-2 Servings.

Ingredients:
3 persimmons, peeled and chopped
¾ cup pomegranate seeds
1 apple, peeled and chopped
10 leaves fresh mint
2 tsp. lemon juice
1 tsp. honey

Directions:
Toss the persimmon, pomegranate seeds, chopped apples, fresh mint, lemon juice, and honey together in a large salad bowl. Allow the ingredients to sit together for about ten minutes before serving to allow the honey and lemon juice to assimilate to the fruits.

GOJI BERRY

Vitamin C is excellent in rejuvenating your immune system and reducing your stress hormone, cortisol. An increased amount of cortisol in your system may cause unnecessary weight gain. Therefore, vitamin C is an essential part of your every day diet. Look to the superfood Goji berry for five hundred times more vitamin C than any orange. Take yourself immediately from stressed to Zen. Also, enjoy the added Goji benefits of vitamin B1, B2, B6, A, and E— perfect for antioxidant cell repair.

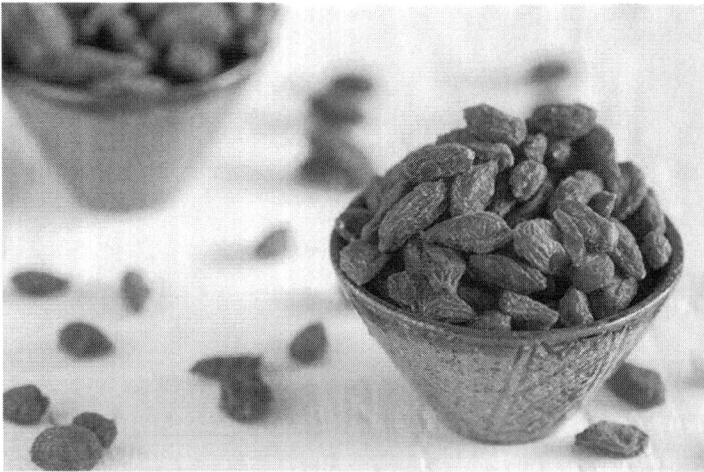

Goji and Bean Fruit Salad

Makes 2-4 Servings.

Ingredients:
2/3 cup sliced almonds
19 ounces chickpeas
10 ounces mandarin orange segments
2/3 cup dried Goji berries
1 diced red onion
1 minced garlic clove
1 inch minced fresh ginger
1 minced jalapeno pepper
1 cup chopped parsley
4 ounces feta cheese, cubed
2 tbsp. apple cider vinegar
2 tbsp. extra virgin olive oil
Black pepper to taste

Directions:
Place a skillet over medium heat with the 2 tbsp. olive oil. Toast the almonds in the olive oil, stirring occasionally. Set them aside after five minutes. Allow them to cool prior to slicing. Prepare your can of chickpeas by rinsing and draining them. Cube your feta cheese to be sprinkled on top of your salad later.

Toss the rinsed chickpeas, mandarin oranges, Goji berries, onion and parsley together with the other 2 tbsp. of olive oil and vinegar in a large salad bowl. Top the salad with the sliced almonds, cubed feta cheese, and salt and pepper to taste. Allow the salad to sit in the refrigerator for three to four hours prior to serving.

Goji-Touting Spring Kale Salad

Makes 2-4 Servings.

Ingredients:
1 cup quinoa
1 large head kale
¾ cup Goji berries
1 cup pine nuts
6 tbsp. olive oil
2 tbsp. apple cider vinegar
2 tsp. Dijon vinegar
2 minced garlic cloves

Directions:
Soak your Goji berries in two cups of water for twenty minutes. Strain the water from the Goji berries afterwards.

Heat a seasoned pan on high and add your pine nuts. Stir quickly; the pine nuts will burn in a matter of minutes. When the pine nuts begin to emit an aroma, take them off the heat.

Prepare your quinoa in two cups of boiling water. Allow it to simmer for fifteen minutes prior to removing it from the heat.

Trim and de-stalk your kale. Slice the kale into ribbons. Place the kale in a large salad bowl.

To the side, whisk your designated dressing: add your lemon juice, Dijon mustard, olive oil, and seasonings.

Add the cooled quinoa to the kale. Toss in the pine nuts and the Goji berries. Coat your salad with your prepared dressing, and enjoy!

ACAI BERRY

Acai berry brings the perfect marriage of chocolate and berry in its amazing flavor. They grow on the Amazonian palm tree and yield several essential fatty acids in their pulp and skin. The essential fatty acids ward off disease and aid in proper brain function, allowing proper communication throughout your neurons.

Acai berries are not eaten whole; instead, it's best to prepare them in salad dressings or glazes for appropriate fatty acid intake. I used Amafruits Acai Puree; it was delicious.

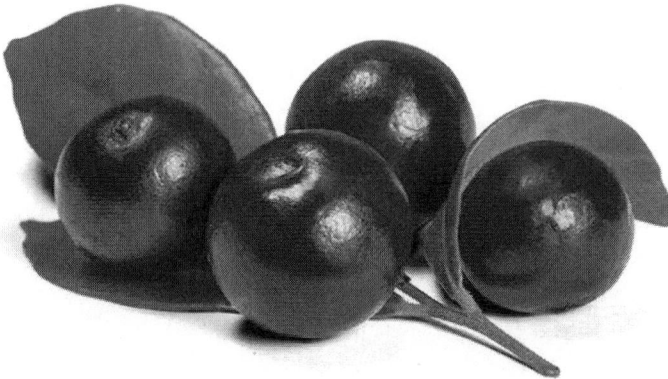

Peppercorn Acai Berry Salad Glaze

Ingredients:
1 pack Amafruits Acai Puree
½ tbsp. Dijon mustard
1 tbsp. balsamic vinegar
1 tbsp. olive oil
Dash of garlic powder
Dash of onion powder
Dash of salt
Dash of cracked peppercorns

Directions:
Whisk your Amafruits Acai Puree together with mustard and vinegar in a medium-sized bowl. Add the olive oil and continue to whisk until the sauce appears creamy. Toss in a dash of salt, onion powder, garlic powder, and cracked peppercorn. Season to taste. Glaze the dressing over your favorite Green Superfood Salad and enjoy!

Acai Berry Glazed Ginger Salad

Makes 2-4 Servings.

Ingredients:
1 ½ cups sliced and cubed honeydew melon
1 ½ cups sliced and cubed cantaloupe
2 peeled and sliced kiwis
1 ½ cups sliced strawberries
½ cups blueberries
3 tbsp. Amafruits Acai Puree
3 tbsp. orange juice
¼ tsp. ground ginger

Directions:
Slice and dice your fruits. Add the honeydew melon, cantaloupe, kiwis, strawberries, and the blueberries to a large bowl. Set it aside.

In a separate, smaller bowl, add the Amafruits Acai Puree, the orange juice, and the ground ginger together and whisk. Add the glaze atop the fruit salad and toss, applying the glaze to the fruits. Enjoy your fibrous fruit salad.

RAW CACAO

Raw Cacao at its most pure level yields the most antioxidants of any known food source in the world. Thus, it is quite good at reducing any cell inflammation while warding off disease. Raw Cacao also contains the much-touted mineral magnesium, which is oftentimes missing from even the most balanced diets.

Raw Cacao Fruit Dipping Sauce

Serves 2.

Ingredients:
2 tbsp. Agave
3 tbsp. Raw Cacao powder
3 tbsp. coconut oil
1/3 tsp. vanilla powder

Directions:
Add the agave, the raw cacao powder, coconut oil, the vanilla powder to a small bowl and mix. Allow the raw cacao powder to fully incorporate with the mixture. Adjust the agave and cacao powder to taste. In order to create a thicker chocolate texture, allow the mixture to sit in the fridge over night. Enjoy the Raw Cacao antioxidant-rich chocolate dip with fiber-rich fruits of your choice!

COCONUTS
AND COCONUT OIL

Coconuts remain the highest source of electrolytes in the world. The water from coconut transports the electrolytes into your blood stream, in turn allowing your body to transport energy from cell to cell. Coconut water has a similar molecular structure to our blood plasma; therefore, your blood cells immediately utilize coconut water as a bloodstream boost.

Coconut Oil contains saturated fats with medium fatty acid chains. Medium fatty acid chains are different than the acid chains in butter and meat—other saturated fat-rich substances. The medium fatty acid chains head straight to the liver and converted into quick energy. Your body begins to burn more calories this way, speeding up your metabolism. Coconut oil has been utilized to ward off and cure diseases in the Pacific Islands for hundreds of years.

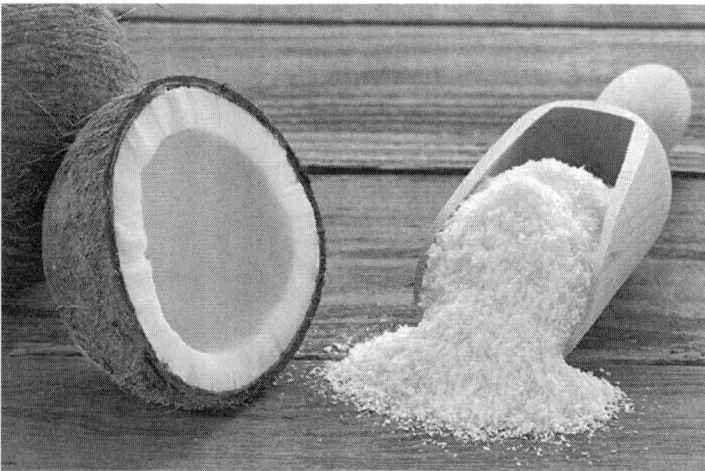

Tropical Coconut Fruit Salad

Makes 2-4 Servings.

Ingredients:
1 peeled and diced papaya
2 peeled and diced mangoes
1 peeled and diced pineapple
2 diced bananas
¼ cup grated coconut

Directions:
Begin by preparing your fruit; peel and slice your papaya, mangoes, diced pineapple, and bananas. Bring the fruit pieces together in a large salad bowl and cover. Allow it to chill in the refrigerator.

Preheat your oven to 350 degrees Fahrenheit and toast your grated coconut for five minutes. Allow them to cool prior to serving atop your juicy fruit salad. Enjoy your electrolyte-rich tropical salad!

Asian-Inspired Coconut Cucumber Summer Salad

Makes 4-6 Servings.

Ingredients:

Dressing:
1/3 cup coconut milk
1 tsp. red curry paste
1 tsp. fish sauce
1 tsp. soy sauce
½ lime's worth of juice
1 tsp. agave
½ tsp. Sriracha

Salad:
½ cup chopped cucumber
½ cup chopped red pepper
½ cup cooked Edamame
½ cup cubed tofu
¼ cup sliced scallions
½ cup chopped basil leaves
5 chopped mint leaves
1 cup arugula
¼ cup toasted coconut flakes

Directions:
Dressing:
Add the dressing ingredients to a small bowl and whisk. If you desire a more thinned-out dressing, add water. Season to taste as you please. Refrigerate as you prepare the salad.

Salad:

Prepare your vegetables: cucumber, red pepper, edamame on the stovetop, scallions, basil leaves, mint leaves, and your arugula. Preheat your oven to 350 degrees Fahrenheit and toast your coconut flakes for ten minutes. Toss the listed salad ingredients—all the vegetables and the tofu and the prepared edamame—in a large salad bowl with the chilled dressing. Add the coconut flakes at the end for a crunchy zest of electrolytes. Enjoy!

NONI FRUIT

Polynesian islanders have looked to the Noni Fruit as medicine for almost two thousand years. Noni works against body bacteria and wards off known killers like E-coli. It strengthens the immune system and works as an antioxidant, reducing cell inflammation. It provides the body with a little extra help by yielding extra vitamins, minerals, enzymes, and phytonutrients.

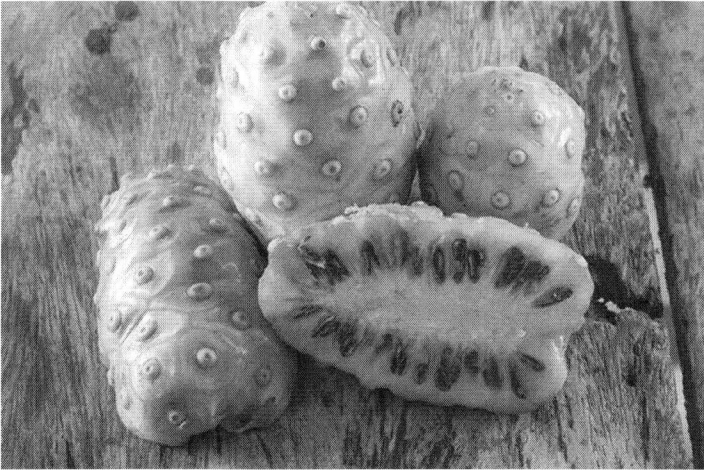

Polynesian Noni Fruit Salad

Makes 2-4 Servings.

Ingredients:
1 cup Noni Juice
1 cup sliced grapes
1 cup peeled and cubed apple
1 cup cubed pineapple
1 cup cherries
1 cup cubed watermelon
2 tbsp. honey
1 tsp. lime juice
1 tsp. lime zest
1 tsp. minced ginger

Directions:
Toss your ingredients into a large salad bowl and mix well. Allow the fruit salad to chill in the refrigerator for about an hour before serving. Indulge in the sweetness and the immune-system boosting effects of this Noni Fruit Salad!

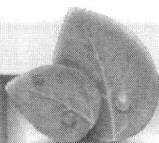

SEEDED SUPERFOOD
SKINNY SALADS

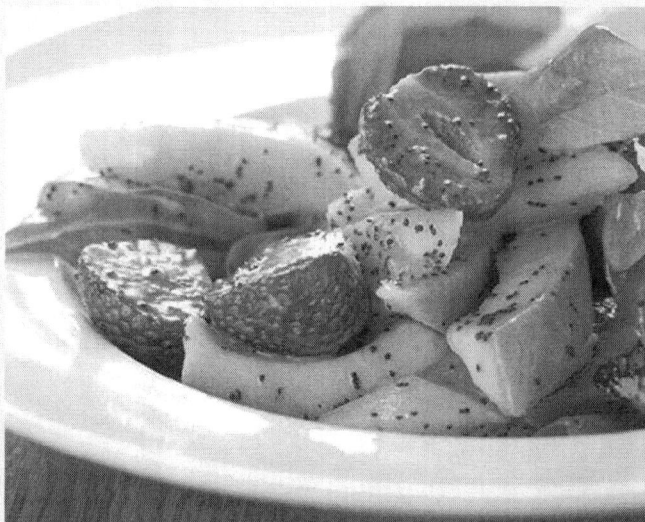

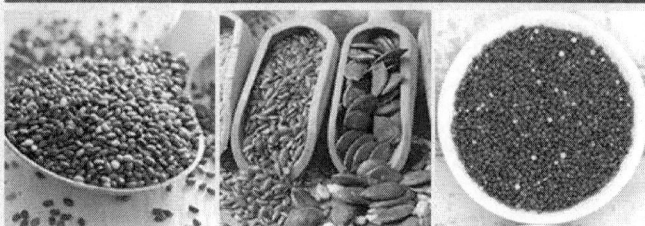

Seed-Based Superfood Skinny Salads

Seeds are often overlooked in the snack-food superfood category as they are incredibly common. Looking at a bag of sunflower seeds, would you imagine their incredible versatility of nutrition and health benefits? Probably not. But a seed is essential for the growth and development of an entire organism. From one, tiny vessel comes a great tree. And that tiny vessel must contain all the nourishment, nutrients, and essential minerals in order to sustain brand new life.

Seed-based superfoods are packed with protein that boosts your metabolism by requiring more calories for digestion. They are the perfect mid-day snack as they provide several anti-inflammatory antioxidants and brain-boosting omega 3 fatty acids.

CHIA SEEDS

The great Aztec warriors looked to the chia seeds for complete survival. The seeds boast eleven grams of fiber per ounce—an incredible half of what you require each day. Chia seeds are filled with omega 3 fatty acids, which allow proper brain communication. Proper brain communication allows regulations of hormones, and regulation of hormones resides in the thyroid gland—the gland responsible for your day-to-day weight regulation. Therefore, the omega 3 fatty acids regulate your weight and allow you to lose weight. It seems like a stretch, but it isn't. Brain communication allows every cell in your body to respond correctly to the food you eat and the environment around you. Furthermore, chia seeds are filled with muscle-building protein that forces your body to utilize more calories to digest, thus revving your metabolism. Chia seeds are also filled with magnesium, iron, zinc, and antioxidants. Chia seeds lend no flavor; therefore, you can add them to any meal and utilize the benefits without halting the other flavors.

Chia-Enriched Kale and Farro Salad

Makes 2-4 Servings.

Ingredients:
1 cup farro
1 large lemon, juiced
3 tbsp. olive oil
4 minced garlic cloves
1 medium shallot
1 tsp. Dijon mustard
2 tbsp. nutritional yeast
1 tsp. freshly ground black pepper
2 tbsp. chia seeds
1 cup chopped green onion
1 cup raw pumpkin seeds
1 cup pomegranate seeds
1 diced pear
5 cups roughly chopped kale

Directions:
Bring the farro to boil in a small saucepan in 2 cups of water, a bit of olive oil, and a pinch of salt. After bringing the farro to a boil, allow it to simmer for about twenty minutes.

To the side, combine your lemon juice, olive oil, minced garlic, shallot, Dijon mustard, and yeast in a food processor. Puree. Next, add the chia seeds to the pureed mixture and stir. The chia seeds will expand in the wet mixture.

Toast your pumpkin seeds in a bit of olive oil over medium heat. They should become brown after approximately five minutes.

Assemble your salad in a large mixing bowl, tossing in the kale, cooked farro, toasted pumpkin seeds, the pomegranate seeds, and the cubed pear. Drizzle with the chia seed dressing and serve!

PUMPKIN SEEDS

Look to your pumpkin-carving clean up to yield some of the best protein-poppers in the land. Pumpkin seeds are also high in iron, zinc, and magnesium. Magnesium works to steady your blood pressure and reduce cortisol in your blood—thus reducing your stress. High stress levels mean weight gain; low stress levels mean weight stabilization and reduction. Pumpkin seeds pack added benefits for men. They yield a high amount of phytosterols that help reduce an enlarged prostate.

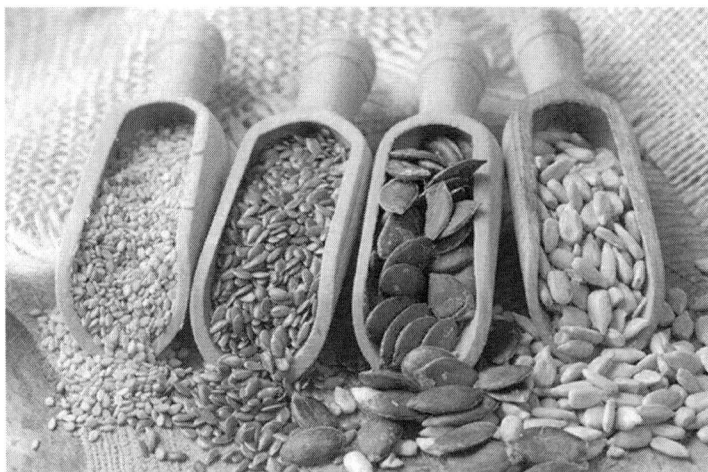

Spicy Pumpkin Seed Salad

Makes 4-6 Servings.

Ingredients:

Dressing:
9 tbsp. olive oil
½ cup diced avocado
½ cup chopped cilantro
¼ cup fresh lime juice
¼ cup toasted and shelled pumpkin seeds
3 tbsp. distilled white vinegar
1 minced garlic clove
¾ tsp. minced Serrano Chile

Salad:
5 ounces spinach
2 halved and sliced avocadoes
12 ounces halved cherry tomatoes
1 diced cucumber
1 sliced jicama
½ sliced onion
1 ½ cup feta cheese
spicy pumpkin seeds

Directions:
To form the avocado-cilantro dressing, add all the ingredients to a blender: olive oil, avocado, cilantro, lime juice, pumpkin seeds, the white vinegar, the garlic, and the Serrano Chile. Blend until the dressing is smooth, not chunky.

Add the spinach to a large salad bowl. Toss in your avocados, tomatoes, cucumber, jicama, and onion. Add the prepared salad dressing and shake, allowing the dressing to form over the mixture. Sprinkle the feta cheese atop the salad along with your spicy pumpkin seeds.

Brown Rice and Pumpkin Seed Salad

Makes 4-6 Servings.

Ingredients:
1 kg cubed pumpkin
2 cups long grain brown rice
1/3 cup pumpkin seed kernels
1/3 cup sunflower seed kernels
1/3 cup lime juice
1 tbsp. soy sauce
½ tsp. sesame oil
1 crushed garlic clove
¼ tsp. brown sugar
1 bunch rocket, torn

Directions:
Begin by baking your pumpkin. Preheat your oven to 400 degrees Fahrenheit and arrange your pumpkin in one layer on your baking sheet. Bake for thirty minutes and set aside.

While the pumpkin bakes in the oven, cook the rice in boiling water for thirty minutes. Set aside to cool, as well.

Change your oven temperature to 350 degrees Fahrenheit and spread your sunflower seeds and pumpkin kernels out in a single layer on a baking tray. Bake for five minutes until browned.

Add the lime juice, soy sauce, sesame oil, garlic, and sugar to a small jar. Shake to create the proper glaze. Pour the prepared long grain brown rice into a large bowl and drizzle it with the lime juice glaze. Stir well. Next, add the rocket, the baked pumpkin, and the baked seeds to the mixture. Stir well and serve immediately!

QUINOA

The marvelous Andes-based superfood Quinoa has been at-large for about five thousand years. Not only does quinoa count as a whole grain seed, supplying your brain with the adequate glucose it needs to process its daily activities; it also works as a complete protein, thus forcing your body to utilize more calories in order to process it. Quinoa is also packed with potassium, magnesium, calcium, and phosphorus.

Summer Black Bean Quinoa Salad

Makes 2-4 Servings.

Ingredients:
1 cup quinoa
2 cups water
¼ cup olive oil
2 juiced limes
2 tsp. ground cumin
1 tsp. salt
½ tsp. red pepper flakes
1 ½ cups halved cherry tomatoes
1 can black beans
5 chopped green onions
¼ cup chopped cilantro
Salt and pepper to taste

Directions:
Bring your quinoa to boil in a medium-sized saucepan.

Reduce the stovetop heat to medium-low, allowing it to simmer beneath a cover. Your quinoa should be tender after around fifteen minutes. Set it aside.

In a medium-sized bowl, whisk your olive oil, lime juice, cumin, salt, and red pepper flakes together.

In a large salad bowl, add your pre-cooked quinoa, tomatoes, black beans, and green onions. Pour the prepared olive oil-based dressing atop the quinoa and black bean mixture. Toss to coat the dressing. Add the chopped cilantro and add salt and pepper to taste. Chill prior to serving.

Quinoa Super Sweet Potato Salad

Makes 4-6 Servings.

Ingredients:
3 cubed sweet potatoes
3 cubed beets
1 chopped head of kale
2 handfuls arugula
1 diced avocado
½ bag thawed peas
2 cups cooked quinoa
2 tbsp. pine nuts
2 tbsp. pumpkin seeds
Salt and pepper to taste

Directions:
Bring four cups of water to a boil in a medium-sized saucepan. Add the 2 cups uncooked quinoa and allow it to cook for about fifteen minutes. Afterwards, the water should be absorbed. Set the quinoa to the side.

Next, you must prepare your sweet potatoes and beets. Chop them and dice them as best as you can. Then, place them in a bag with a bit of olive oil. Shake to coat the vegetables. Spread the beets and sweet potatoes out on the baking sheet and cook at 400 degrees Fahrenheit for forty minutes. Be sure to flip the vegetables halfway through the cook session.

Assemble your salad in a large salad bowl. Add your baked sweet potatoes and beets, your head of kale, your arugula, and your thawed peas. Toss in your cooked quinoa, avocado, pine nuts, and your pumpkin seeds as well. Be sure to mix the salad. Add salt and pepper to taste.

Feta Cheese Mediterranean Quinoa Salad

Makes 2-4 Servings.

Ingredients

Vinaigrette:
3 tbsp. lemon juice
1 tbsp. red wine vinegar
¼ tsp. oregano
1 crushed garlic clove
Salt and pepper to taste
¼ cup olive oil

Salad:
1 cup quinoa
Salt and pepper to taste
2 cups halved grape tomatoes
1 cup black olives
3 sliced onions
2 diced pickled cherry peppers
½ diced cucumber
1 cup sprinkled feta

Directions:
To form the vinaigrette, whisk the lemon juice, vinegar, oregano, garlic and salt and pepper together in a small bowl. Add the olive oil in a slow pour. Allow it to sit together.

Boil the quinoa for about fifteen minutes, covered, prior to removing it from the heat and allowing it to cool.

Add the cooled quinoa to a large salad bowl. Toss in the tomatoes, olives, onions, cherry peppers, cucumbers, and prepared dressing. Allow the dressing to coat the mixture. Leave the salad to cool in the refrigerator for up to eight hours. The flavor increases with time. Sprinkle with feta cheese and serve!

SUNFLOWER SEEDS

Sunflower seeds protect your skin from aging. Just a few handfuls a day provide all your required alpha-tocopherol for the day. Alpha-tocorpherol is an active ingredient in Vitamin E. It protects your cells from powerful radiation.

Furthermore, these tiny morsels contain heaps of phnylalanine, a natural antidepressant. Phenylalanine reconfigures to norepinephrine in the brain, allowing you to stay in the moment, ready for anything.

Johnny Apple and Sunflower Seed Spring Salad

Makes 2-4 Servings.

Ingredients:
2 cubed green apples
½ cup sunflower seeds
1 chopped head romaine lettuce
2 diced dill pickles
2 diced tomatoes

Directions:
Prepare your fruit, romaine lettuce, dill pickles, and tomatoes. Add them to a large salad bowl. Pour your sunflower seeds in with the mixture. Toss in your choice of salad dressing—may I suggest one of the many superfood dressings included in this recipe book!

Sunflower Grape Salad

Makes 2-4 Servings.

Ingredients:
3 tbsp. red wine vinegar
1 tsp. honey
1 tsp. maple syrup
½ tsp. mustard
2 tsp. grapeseed oil
7 cups arugula
2 cups halved red grapes
2 tbsp. toasted sunflower seed kernels
1 tsp. chopped thyme
¼ tsp. salt
¼ tsp. pepper

Directions:
Pour vinegar, honey, syrup, and mustard into a small bowl. Add the oil slowly, whisking the dressing together.

Toast the shelled sunflower seeds in a preheated 350 degree Fahrenheit oven for five minutes. Allow them to cool prior to serving with the salad.

Add the arugula, halved grapes, toasted seeds, and the thyme in a large salad bowl. Toss the salad in the prepared dressing. Enjoy!

HEMP SEEDS

Hemp seeds are filled with essential fatty acids, beneficial for brain function. Furthermore, hemp seeds deliver a great amount of protein. They contain all nine essential amino acids. By making hemp seeds a part of your daily diet you decrease your of diabetes risk by fifty percent as the magnesium content increases insulin sensitivity in your blood. Therefore, hemp seeds are excellent weight-loss tools: increased insulin sensitivity allows you to understand when you need food and when you don't.

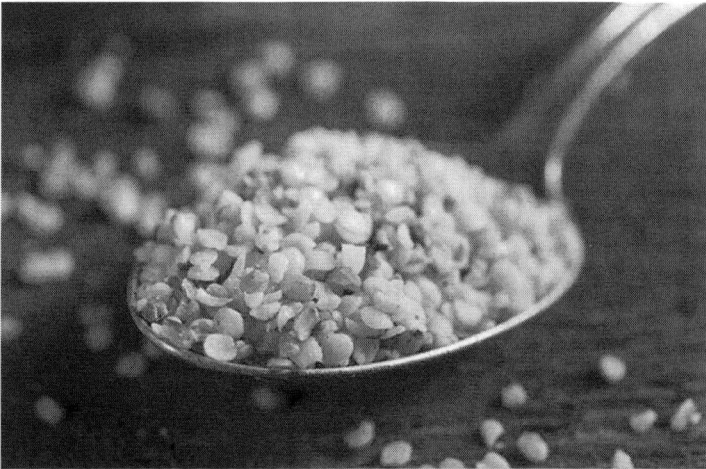

Tabbouleh and Hemp seed Salad

Makes 2-4 Servings.

Ingredients:
1 bunch chopped parsley
2 cups diced cucumber
1 cup diced tomato
¾ cup diced red bell pepper
¼ cup diced onion
½ cup Nutiva Organic Hemp seed
¼ cup lemon juice
2 minced garlic cloves
6 tbsp. Nutiva Organic Hemp Oil
1 tsp. salt

Directions:
Prepare your parsley by chopping it and tossing it into a large salad bowl. Slice and dice the rest of your vegetables: cucumber, tomato, red pepper, and your onion. Add these to the large salad bowl as well. Follow the vegetables with the hemp seeds.

On the side, add the lemon juice, garlic, hemp oil, and salt into a blender. Blend until you achieve a smooth consistency.

Pour the prepared dressing overtop the vegetable and hemp salad. Toss to coat the vegetables with the hemp-laden, protein-rich dressing. Enjoy!

Summer Picnic Hempseed Salad

Makes 2-4 Servings.

Ingredients:
2 tbsp. red wine vinegar
1 tbsp. olive oil
2 diced tomatoes
1 sliced cucumber
2 tbsp. olives
1 tbsp. oregano
Handful of spinach
3 tbsp. hempseeds
Salt and pepper to taste

Directions:
In a large salad bowl, add your vinegar and then add the olive oil in a slow pour, whisking steadily. Next, add diced tomatoes, sliced cucumbers, olives, oregano, spinach, hempseeds, and your salt and pepper to taste. Toss the salad prior to serving. Enjoy!

Conclusion

Superfood salad recipes yield essential nutrients, antioxidants and proteins needed for optimal health without counteracting any flavor. Each salad creates a textured, intense experience—one that leaves you searching for future nourishment in the form of other superfoods to fuel your lifestyle. Once you have discovered the benefits the world provides in these tiny seeds, in these leaf-like vegetables, and in these vibrant, colorful fruits—you won't want to return to your preservative rich lifestyle.

You'll be swimming with the benefits: your brain will be honed with the proper cell-to-cell communication contributed by the omega 3 fatty acids in the seeds. Your cell inflammation will have reduced immensely from the antioxidants. And your waist will have diminished. Weight loss is an added benefit to supplementing your healthy lifestyle with these immaculate food choices. The world of superfoods will provide you with the medicine you need to survive and thrive!

Printed in Great Britain
by Amazon.co.uk, Ltd.,
Marston Gate.